MEDITATION

MEDITATION

Good For You

Translated by Carla R. Mancari

Celestial Literary Group

The contents of this book are not meant to take the place of qualified medical professionals or therapists. There is no expressed or implied guarantee as to the effects of the suggestions given or the liability taken.

Contents

Acknowledgments

Sincere thanks to Mary Carpenter, who reviewed and edited the manuscript. Her dedication is appreciated.

With the most profound love, I am grateful for the gift of the Minute Meditation.

Introduction

From its conception, the Minute Meditation has helped individuals from all walks of life. For more than forty-five years, I have taught individuals and groups meditation. During this time, I began to observe that those who chose to practice one minute twice a day were realizing balance and contentment in their daily lives — all direct benefits of meditation.

It became apparent that those individuals with limited time could benefit from meditation that was supported by an awareness of the Spiritual Center. The Minute Meditation offers a means of quickly and easily accessing your Spiritual Center. The Minute Meditation is a secular practice available for you who wish to learn to meditate and travel a direct path to your Spiritual Center, allowing you to make the necessary life change.

The humorous stories included are either ones that I have written or that I have heard many times on my life's journey from many different teachers, masters, and gurus. Therefore, it's not possible to assign credit to any particular individual for the originality.

1

WHY
LEARN TO MEDITATE?
Something Missing

Why learn to meditate? A silent meditation practice may softly guide you to where you may access your Spiritual Center (chapter 5). The ultimate work of meditation practice is to transform your life into a more balanced and contented life. As a contributing human being in a busy world, you may always be striving to be accomplished. Still, something is missing. What is it?

Intellectually you know there must be something missing in your life. You may want to believe that your spirituality is realized in intellectual teachings from which you may achieve a temporary emotional high. Yes, but an emotional high is a temporary fix.

It's easy to get lost in a world that gives you a high one day and a low the next. Worldly wisdom or intellectual pursuits may temporarily satisfy, but they leave you without the aware presence of your life. That is what is missing.

For you to intentionally or unintentionally seek the different metaphysical teachings to realize what is missing may stimulate your mind and cause you to feel uplifted. You would continuously be rising to the mental state of consciousness, and the mind tends to keep you where it feels good. Your seeking to reach your full potential based on outer pursuits is like the miner who is easily attracted to fool's gold. You may become content to fulfill your quest by only seeking what glitters. It may be shiny and may look like the real thing, but the real thing it is not.

There is nowhere out here that you can realize what is missing. It's the mind's work to want to take you on an outer journey. That is what the mind does best. Meditation takes you on an inner journey to what may be missing. It is all about an inner journey, a journey that begins not out here, but within you.

Why learn to meditate? Meditation practice is a vehicle that delivers you to your destination. Meditation practice may endow you with a greater awareness of an inner path that acknowledges your spirituality. You may connect with your root being.

You may become aware that you are more than a name. You are more than an individual who walks this earth. Yours is more than the physical sense of the life of which you are so guarded and protective. Yours is a spiritual nature.

Perhaps you have a strong opposition to a constant reminder that you have a greater reality. But you cannot separate yourself from that which you are. Learn to meditate and awaken to the good news that there is more.

Meditation guides your footsteps directly to the silence of awareness of your Spiritual Center (chapter 5). You are all that is necessary. You have the necessary wherewithal to accomplish whatever is required of you to realize your full potential.

You live at a time and in a world where many choices are presented. Meditation is one of them. Why not take a direct inner path? Why not say yes to a meditation that requires no intermediary.

You are all that is necessary to accomplish whatever it is you may seek to realize. When you consent and awaken to the spirituality of your inner source, the unreal may recede. Your spirituality may continuously be revealed within your Spiritual Center.

2

WHY IT'S GOOD FOR YOU

Taking Out The Trash

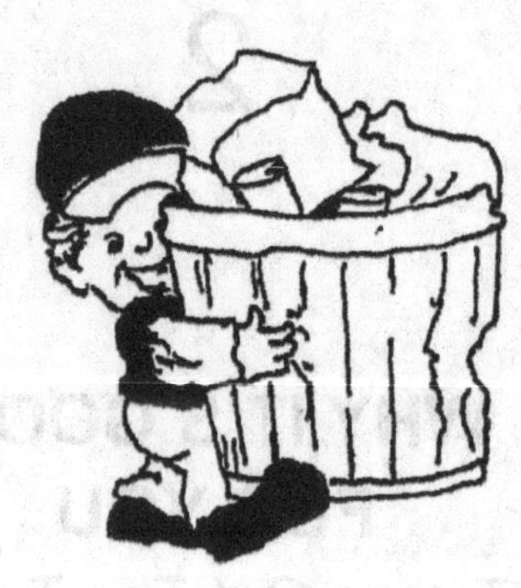

Are you taking out the trash or taking it in? If trash comes to your door, do you open it and invite it in? That is an easy one—your answer would likely be, "Of course not."

Well, how about when you are confronted with negativity? Do you allow your mind to absorb it? How does meditation help you with the answer to this one? Two words: interior cleansing.

A meditation practice may be simple. There may be no lengthy-time requirements, no prescribed rituals, and no use of a word, thought, image, sound, or breath. Therefore, you may be inclined to believe it can't deliver what it promises.

You may ask, "What exactly is happening when I meditate? What is going on when I don't dialogue, return to my Spiritual Center area, and rest with awareness? What could possibly be occurring that could benefit me?"

The answers are conditioning awareness, internal cleansing, and the realization of your spirituality. All of which contribute to a life change and the ability to fulfill your life's potential. That is what may be occurring.

CONDITIONING

Your consciousness is vibrating energy. Through negative thought, word, or deed you may misuse or pollute the purest of your vibrating energy. From the moment you enter this world until you leave it, your consciousness is affected by positive and negative conditioning. Conditioning is accomplished through the labels, names, or identities given to individuals and objects by repetition.

Your sense of your mind and your physical body are given a name. The repetition of your given name causes you to identify with it as who you are. You are taught the use of "I," "me," "my," and "mine," to which you become attached. All are concepts—none of which are who you are.

As an aware, conscious being, you have a mind and thoughts; and through your body's organs, you receive impressions from your senses—sight, hearing, smell, taste, touch—that are stamped with the conditioning of the society in which you live. Conditioning is continually being taught or passed on by parents, friends, peers, and authority figures. Your moral judgment is based on the conditioning of that which is considered to be "right" or "wrong" according to tradition, culture or religion.

Because an object is constructed for use, you are conditioned to think and see the object's practical use rather than to realize its essence. For example, a block of wood that is cut from a tree and then carved into a chair or table is always seen and thought of as a chair or table. But actually, it is still the wood, and if it were burned it would be ash.

The chair or table is a functional concept of its reality. You aren't aware of purely seeing. You see a concept. If you aren't an aware being, you believe in the conditioned sense impressions. This also applies to your form and your spirituality.

Conditioning does create useful functional concepts that serve to identify objects and individuals. However, it also may create false concepts of thought patterns and sense impressions. False concepts are created when you accept the *appearance* of anything or any individual as their reality.

The complete conditioning of the mind, thoughts, and the physical body is a collection of sense impressions that lead you to falsely identify as a separate personal being. Thus, even though you are not a separate personal being, your every thought, word, and action is designed to protect this false identity, which results in the misuse of your vibrating energy. Of course, it's necessary to use conceptual terms to communicate in this world.

It is the misuse of your individual expression of consciousness that is a problem, and this expression must be restored to its original purity. A meditation practice helps to purify your vibrating energy with the least amount of

time and effort. To realize your spirituality is to be free to express your full
potential.

INTERIOR CLEANSING

Interior cleansing is a purification
and forgiveness process. To puri-
fy/forgive is to cleanse any of your
misused, negative vibrating energy.
The prefix "for" translates as away,
apart, and off. One of the definitions of
"give" is to inflict punishment. So, to
"for"-"give" is to do away with, not to
inflict punishment. Forgiveness is secular. It covers you and everyone who
may come to mind. It's a gift of your
nature, which may be given freely and
which causes no harm.

You may say, "I can forgive, but I
can never forget." You can't talk about
forgiving without talking about forgetting. True forgiveness *is* forgetting, let-
ting go, doing away with. To be attached to the "not forgetting" is to de-

prive yourself of the vibrating energy that exists for your use.

You cannot accept *more* while you are holding onto *less.* Attachment binds you to this world and limits your freedom of being. The belief that "you" exist as a separate person allows attachment to come into existence.

In your spirituality, there isn't a time when you aren't at one with your inner source. The moment you think "I, me, my, mine," attachment arises, and that causes suffering. It's the false belief in a personal sense that causes unreal experiences of an imaginary, separate self. It is a self who is disruptive, defensive, and oversensitive, with a desire to please everyone and is in constant search for approval.

Your false concept of a personal self creates a life that perpetuates false concepts. Attachment of any kind is the misuse of energy. Thoughts in and of themselves have no emotions attached to them. You attach your descriptive judgment of "good," "bad," "hurtful," or "pleasurable" to them.

The attachment to pleasure can be a subtle pull in its direction. Interestingly, there are seldom, if ever, any complaints about the emotions that give pleasure; however, the rising energy is the same. One thought is no different from another. Vibrating energy is vibrating energy.

The emotional differences that you attach to your thoughts are based on your conditioned memory experiences. To attach hate, anger, joy, love to thoughts that rise one moment and fall the next is to attach falsely to that which cannot sustain itself. The Minute Meditation practice teaches you the discipline of not dialoguing with thoughts, sensations, or emotions. This paves the way for the detachment of the thoughts, sensations, or emotions without strenuous practices or effort.

To become detached doesn't mean that you are indifferent or aloof; instead, you find yourself merely aware of the thoughts, sensations, and various states and levels of consciousness that rise and fall throughout the day. You realize you have the power to attach—or not to attach—emotions to each of these. Here is the priceless value of meditation practice: once there is no longer a response to a negative thought, it ceases suffering. When your hurts and sufferings arise during meditation practice, you create a space between not-dialoguing. In that space, an "instant" of purification occurs.

It's an "instant" that cannot be felt or emotionally experienced. Feeling is of the mind, and the purification "instant" is beyond the mind. What you may realize is the result. Each time you respond to the hurtful memories during your daily life experiences by dialoguing, you are reliving the event and thus multiplying your suffering. But the purification "instant" during a meditation practice may do away with an entire history of multiplied hurts.

You realize purification has taken place when the same hurtful memory rises again, and *you are no longer negatively affected.* Purification doesn't mean you will no longer remember. Your memory remains intact, but the suffering attached to the memory no longer exists.

You come into the forgetting of the suffering—and then you realize, "I can forgive and forget." What value can you place on that? It is life-changing, your life, your suffering.

As you turn inward to practice meditation, it brings a realization of your spirituality with the least amount of time and effort. The internal cleansing and purification process intensifies and speeds up; your vibrating energy is restored; your words, thoughts, and deeds are no longer misguided or distorted. An "instant" of silence during the purification process is profound. It's an internal cleansing of your individual consciousness's vibrating negative energy, restoring it to its original pure state. Because meditation is a direct, subtle, and calming practice, it connects to your inner power, where an "instant" of purification may occur.

Think about how easy it is for you to attach emotions to thoughts immediately. Think about how fickle the mind is and how quickly you become caught up in it. You have a choice to suffer or not—a choice of forgiving and forgetting. How life-changing is that?

Meditation supports a steady movement of the internal cleansing process. You may experience a sudden release of tears of joy. You may find you seek silence, tend to speak less, and listen more.

Healing old hurts, being free from memories' attachments, enjoying a more significant amount of joy, and opening the door where silence pervades—these are among the many benefits of the cleansing process. It is a necessary beginning during meditation practice. Internal cleansing bears the most delectable fruit. It brings the most beautiful peace: a pliable peace that permeates your entire being and is expressed in all that you are and do.

3

BALANCE
Slow Down

Why is it essential that you learn to meditate? Well, when your life has a feel of tipsy, it may be that you are trying to pull yourself in different directions. There may be times when you are trying to balance your life's consciousness, mind, and body. It may cause you to come crashing down. Meditation may help you to lead a balanced life.

Concerns for your physical, emotional and financial well-being; a sense of responsibilities; and change may contribute to a lack of balance. To balance your life, slow down, meditate, ponder, do less, and enjoy what you do. It is better to do a few things that you enjoy than many that you do from old habits or obligations. Balance comes from being aware when to sit still, when to stay in place, and when to move about in a quiet, steady motion.

Take time for meditation, and you may find the insights that are necessary for you to live a balanced life is within your grasp. Time is not your enemy. It is a tool that you use. It is what you share with yourself and others. Remember to share it with yourself and use it wisely. The rat race is for rats, don't join it.

4

STRESSED
Overworked

Stress is another good reason for meditation practice. There may be times when you feel put upon by others. There may be times when the position you are in tests your ability to say "enough."

There is such a thing as being too responsible. Wanting to do all that is demanded of you is not always possible. Admitting this to yourself and finally to those who make the demands, may be a challenge you find difficult. The earth plane limits you by time and space. It has laws that you must respect and obey. When you do not, stress is one of the consequences.

You are manifesting upon this earth plane as mental and physical states of consciousness. Neglect or stress abuses the mental and physical form that you are using. You are the caretaker; and the mental and physical form reacts to the care, negative or positive, that you give it.

Your mental and physical form only has you to stand up for it. They only have you to safeguard them from the many demands the world would make of them. You are not a super person. You are not a workhorse. Overworking your mental and physical states of consciousness is an accident waiting to happen.

If you cannot take charge of your mental and physical well being, others will do it for you; unfortunately, not for the betterment of your well-being. You are not here to do all things or to be all things in whatever position you find yourself. Reflect carefully; a meditation practice may help you to better make the necessary decisions for the protection of your mind and body. Get your priorities straight. Your mental and physical health needs an adversary; meditation can be that adversary.

5

The Spiritual Center
An Invitation

There is an old story that goes something like this: After God had created humankind, God called one of the angels and asked the angel to hide the one thing God wished to conceal.

"I have finished except for one thing: the mystery of life. Where shall you hide it?" God asked the angel.

"I will hide it in outer space," responded the excited angel.

"No," God said, *"one day, someone will easily find it there."*

"All right, I will hide it on the moon. Surely it will not be found there?"

"No, no," said God, *"one day, they will be able to look there also. Hmmm, I have it! Let's put it within them. They would never think to look there!"*

There is a gentle, subtle vibrating center within you (in the center of the chest, between the breasts). It's called the Spiritual Center. The Spiritual Center is well known in the East as the Fourth Chakra, Anahata Chakra.

Although often written about and discussed, the Spiritual Center's direct availability and easy access are *often* ignored. It is the most neglected entrance into the inner sanctuary of your being. There are seven spiritual centers (chakras) within the physical body. They begin at the base of the spine and end at the top of the head. These vibrating energy centers are located three below the Spiritual Center and three above it. The Spiritual Center is the powerhouse that influences the centers above and below it.

This pure vibrating energy center does not have a particular religious affiliation. Members from any religion, or none, may access it. The Spiritual Center is the connection to all states and levels of consciousness. And depending on the state of consciousness you choose to realize — Buddha, Hindu, Christ, or any other — then, that is the one you may realize. It is amazing!

It is here beyond all religions that mystical mysteries are resolved. Where knowledge, understanding, insights, and wisdom reside. It is here that your spirituality is realized. Most importantly, with the help of meditation, resolutions are born in moments of critical situations, and the answers needed in your practical life may come forth.

Though this powerful energy center is within you, it may seem strange and unfamiliar; you may shy away from this vital center from fear of the unknown. It may require courage for you to venture beyond the known into the depths of your Spiritual Center. You may prefer to stick with what you believe you know.

Fortunately, meditation gently guides you to the point where you may access your Spiritual Center. This is your birthright and may be reflected in your daily living. Meditation continuously connects you with your Spiritual Center in the Oneness of love. The unconditional love of your Spiritual Center may guide you through your daily activities.

Every individual, every creature, is a loving expression of the Oneness of unconditional love. The one who tills the soil, the one who plants the seed, the one who encourages the growth, the one who gathers the crops, the one who packages it, ships it, stocks it, and the one who brings the banquet to the table for your nourishment: all are expressions of the unconditional love that nurtures the universe. You cannot eat a meal without being aware that the least upon the table is an expression of that unconditional love.

During a meditation practice, with the awareness of your Spiritual Center, you may realize an unconditional love that has a natural ability to include, embrace, and permeate all individual beings. It gives all to all and holds back nothing from those who are aware and receptive. When you rest with the silent awareness of your Spiritual Center area, you possess the natural inclination to share this kind of love, and it is in the sharing of it that you come into the aware and receptive awareness of *your* unconditional loving nature. It is a nature that is aware it is in giving back that is the foundation of a contented, full life.

Look in the least expected place: within you. There you may bask with the silent awareness of your Spiritual Center. The Spiritual Center invites and beckons you now to go within so that you may realize what is yours. It does not matter how isolated you may have felt in the past; the radiant light of your Spiritual Center will hold you in unconditional love.

All the strength and action you could ever desire in your life exist in every vibration of your Spiritual Center. The vibrating energy is invulnerable power that may dissipate sorrowful remorse, soothe a troubled mind, and restore relationships. The Spiritual Center may guide your footsteps to an awareness of your inherent spirituality. Here you may become aware of your uniqueness as an individual expression of consciousness. You may become aware of this power as you practice meditation.

This power radiates a light that you may step into and with which you may be as one as you rest with silent awareness of your Spiritual Center. Your spiritual power is a center of compassion, clarity, discernment, and wisdom. You may become aware that, indeed, less of this world is more, and more of this world is not necessary.

The power to wash away greed and bathe you in total love resides in your Spiritual Center. The power of love is without limits, and it cannot be diminished. It is a protective strength and eternal grace that accompanies you constantly on your life's journey and envelops your conscious mind.

You may have been led to believe that the conscious mind is the power to be harnessed. Yes, the mind is a powerful instrument, and when it is focused on the things of this world, it may perform seemingly magical feats and fulfill desires. But the mind, in and of itself, has no power. All it can do is what is given to it from within.

The mind may manifest desired attractions, but it may also cause mischief and create obstacles where there are none. To work only with the mind is to deny yourself the opportunity to go beyond the mind to where the power exists, your Spiritual Center. The power is given directly to you from within. You decide whether to invest the power in the manifestations of attractions in this world. You may use or misuse your power of vibrating energy.

If you choose to build your life with a thought-focused mind, you are building on quicksand. Attractions created by thoughts follow the path of thoughts: they rise, they fall. The mind left to its own devices is easily distracted. A thought-focused mind is an attempt to realize your potential by force, which is not possible! The peace, joy, and comfort you seek exist not within the mind, but within your Spiritual Center.

With meditation practice, you may realize the power within and hear the silence. You may realize that with this silence, awareness of your Spiritual Center area is readily available to you. Here you may bask in the vibrating energy of consciousness. It is from here that whatever is necessary to meet your needs manifests without relying on the mind's creations.

Become aware of the power within your Spiritual Center. This essential power dissolves the darkness created by ignorance and the fear that darkness breeds. Become aware of a quiet that is only available when you regularly connect with the power of your Spiritual Center.

No code, no secret password, no referral, and no formal introduction is needed for you to meet and access your Spiritual Center. It will never be enough for you just to know about your Spiritual Center. You will always long to connect to and access it. *The Minute Meditation* is the boat that will carry you across the river into your Spiritual Center. Get in and take the ride of your life, which will take you to a new beginning of you.

6

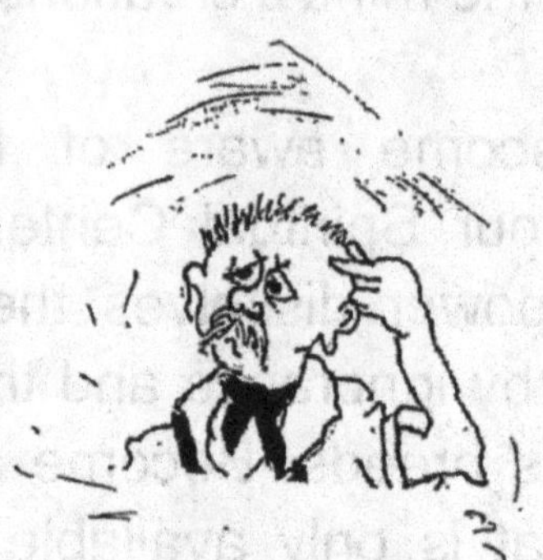

The Minute Meditation
Revelation

How confused are you? Do the many different contemplation, meditation, and concentration practices have you confused? Is there a meditation that can help you to become a more aware individual? A meditation without all of the time and energy consumption required? Yes, there is. It's the Minute Meditation.

The Minute Meditation (also known as M&M, because it is sooo sweet to you) is a revealed life-changing meditation of awareness that may allow you to realize your full potential. It is a minute of infinite power. It is a minute of profound rest. It is a subtle, calming minute that allows you to move effortlessly to the silent awareness of your Spiritual Center area. It is the gift that keeps on giving.

The Minute Meditation drops the more traditional aids—such as a word, thought, image, sound, or breath—and articulates simplicity. The Minute Meditation also drops the traditionally extended periods, rigid posture, and strict rules of other practice regimens. The Minute Meditation intends to establish you firmly in your spirituality. Your life is built upon hallowed ground and is rooted in love. The Minute Meditation connects you to the awareness of this hallowed ground so that you can accept your inner guidance and realize your full potential.

The Minute Meditation provides a means for your inherent "image and likeness" to be restored to its full stature. It supports, strengthens, and deepens your ongoing connection with your Spiritual Center. Without extraneous dialogue, stringent guidelines, or complicated definitions, the Minute Meditation bypasses the potential distractions in which the mind loves to indulge.

The Minute Meditation is a practice of "undoing." You are being guided to undo many years of conditioning with the least amount of effort. It is the opposite of what you have been taught in modern culture.

You have been conditioned that to accomplish whatever it is you want, you must "do"—sometimes overdo—to achieve your goal. You push, shove, and drive yourself to the brink to get what it is you believe you want. Getting and grasping; effort, effort, all is an effort. The Minute Meditation teaches you to do the opposite. Relax. There is no pushing, no shoving, and no driving yourself anywhere. You simply rest with the silence of awareness of your Spiritual Center area for one minute, twice a day. Force and exertion are not necessary. You may receive what you need when you release and let go of the driving pressure.

The most significant effort that you can expend is to show up and be patient for one minute, twice a day. With the silent awareness of your Spiritual Center area, a minute is an eternity. The mind takes you on an

outer journey through the alluring attractions of this world. The Minute
Meditation takes you on a direct inner
journey through the aware spirituality
of your nature. When faithfully practiced, the Minute Meditation slowly,
carefully, and lovingly connects your
inner reality to your outer physical life.

A lack of understanding of your
reality creates distortions. Presently
you are working with conventional
mind-body consciousness and the
perception of a false sense of a separate self. The Minute Meditation allows
you to venture beyond the usual
mindset into a sense of your reality
with awareness. The Minute Meditation establishes you in the unconditional, nonjudgmental truth that dwells
naturally in your Spiritual Center.

Your nature has many facets.
Within your Spiritual Center, the brilliance of your inner power is continuously revealing its light. When you let
go and are willing to embrace yet an-

other previously unknown facet of your nature, the life-changing transition is welcomed. The Minute Meditation is a meditation practice for those who have an interest in learning to meditate in solitude, simplicity, and silence for one minute twice a day. It is a path to the awareness of your indwelling Spiritual Center. The Minute Meditation may connect you with infinite power and profound rest.

All silent meditations may have their value. What is it specifically that makes the Minute Meditation life-changing? This silent practice eliminates the middleman—the breath, word, sound, or thought. It is a short, direct path that guides you, without interference or obstacles, to the awareness of your Spiritual Center area. Nothing needs to stand between you and your reality. The Minute Meditation may cut to the chase in leading you to realize your full potential.

The Minute Meditation may require some adjustment of your ideas concerning what "ought" to happen. But the deep silence this practice generates will more than reward your attitude adjustment. Yes, less *is* more. When you begin the Minute Meditation, you respond to the invitation to come home. You are accepting your inner guidance.

The structures of the world, no matter their magnitude, will not endure. Your enduring structure is your Spiritual Center. Through the Minute Meditation practice, you learn to no longer place your trust in the things of this world which come and go. You no longer choose to erect frameworks that separate you from your reality. You choose the life-changing reality of your true nature.

The Minute Meditation's inward pilgrimage of the unknown may take you to the knowledge of inner peace. You come to realize that this peace is a resting silence within your being. Learn to meditate with the Minute Meditation. This time-honored practice is a revelation for a generation whose time has come and who *is* ready to receive. There is a presence with the awareness of your Spiritual Center area that the world cannot comprehend. Seek it. Go for it!

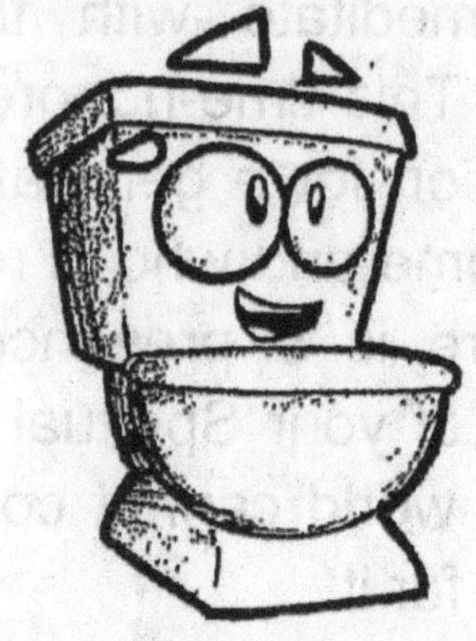

7

The Practice
Three Easy Steps

How many motivational speakers must you listen to and how often must you listen in order to be motivated? Why look to others to lift your spirit and move you to realize your full potential? Your Spiritual Center *is* the greatest motivational speaker. The Minute Meditation of awareness practice may ground and balance you during your daily activities.

The Minute Meditation is an easy meditation of awareness practice that you may learn quickly. Sit comfortably on a couch or chair; sitting on the floor is optional. If your health does not permit you to practice in a sitting position, you may lie down.

The Minute Meditation may be practiced at any time before a meal, at least two hours after a meal, or about an hour after drinking juice (the changing energy vibration will interfere with the digestion process). Water is fine. Over time, you will find that your inner practice moves in the direction of a minimum amount of effort. *A word of CAUTION:* Never practice any form of contemplation, quiet time, meditation, or awareness, even for a moment, while driving, operating machinery, or at any time when your safety may be at risk.

THE PRACTICE:

1. Sit comfortably, rest your hands in your lap or by your sides, and close your eyes. Next, slowly and deeply inhale; then very slowly exhale, relaxing your entire body. Then continue to breathe normally.

2. Consciously become aware of your Spiritual Center *area* (center of your chest, between the breasts) and rest with the silence of awareness.

3. When thoughts or sensations arise, do not dialogue, converse, engage, or respond to their rising. Your attention is already there. Allow them to be, then return again to your Spiritual Center *area* and rest with the silence of awareness.

That's it. Is that easy enough? It's this simple, silent, one-minute, twice-a-day practice that may help you quickly reap all your inherent benefits to realizing your full potential. At the end of a practice period, take a moment to become consciously aware of your mental and physical senses again before returning to your normal activities.

~~

Listen to what an individual who has taken the Minute Meditation challenge has to say about it:

Grahame, a retired postman in Australia, reports on his practice:

Spending just one minute twice a day out of my busy routine does wonders for me. Whenever I feel overwhelmed by the stress of modern living, I take one minute to put it right.

I sit quietly, take a deep breath, and I bring my awareness to the center of my chest, my heart center. I allow my awareness to be with this area just resting but staying alert.

Just one minute twice a day with this practice alleviates tension, and I feel rejuvenated with a new perspective.

The Minute Meditation practice allows me to function back in the crazy world with a new wholeness and vitality. It has brought peace and assurance in my life that I thought not possible. I'm grateful.

~~

Recurring comments from practitioners of the Minute Meditation:

- I sleep better.

- I'm less prone to harbor resentments.

- My children tell me I'm easier to get along with.

- I'm more flexible when things don't go my way.

- I experience more joy in my life and more self-acceptance.

- I'm happier, and my friends say, "You're nicer to be around."

- My emotional responses to life's ups and downs are more appropriate and less exaggerated.

~~

In coming home to themselves at the deepest level, Minute Meditation practitioners report an ability to remember what their lives are all about. By effortlessly resting in the silent awareness of their Spiritual Center area for just one minute, twice a day, many people state that they return to their daily activities with renewed energy and a new sense of purpose. The comment most often made is, "It changed my life." Such reports are indeed an incentive to take up the life-changing Minute Meditation practice and reap its benefits.

Each time that thoughts, emotions, or any of the senses (sight, hearing, smell, taste, touch) seek your attention, gently again become aware of your Spiritual Center area. Repeating the practice, again and again, is not starting over, beginning again, or going backward—it *is* continuing. Do not label or dialogue internally with any of the thoughts, emotions, or senses that may arise within a practice period. All thoughts, sensations, and images will fall away if you do not engage with them. For an instant, you may rest with silent awareness.

Be consistent with your practice: one minute, twice a day. Do it. To say "I'll try" builds in failure. To *do* assures the possibility of success. Success may come by doing. Trying gives you a way out. Doing gives you a way in; into all that you seek to realize — your full potential.

If, for any reason, you find it challenging to become aware of your Spiritual Center *area,* place your hand upon your Spiritual Center area (center of your chest, between the breasts) for the first few practice periods. You are not seeking to feel anything. The mind feels. You are resting in the silence of awareness beyond mind-body consciousness.

Be aware that thoughts, emotions, and sense impressions *will rise* in mind during your practice. This is what the mind does: it thinks. That is its purpose. You are not practicing to stop or still the mind. You are choosing to not *dialogue* with the thoughts, and to create the opportunity for purification.

Once purified, a memory or sense impression will never plague you again. The energy you would have expended on the memory or sense-impression is now available for you to consciously decide how to use. Be kind and loving with yourself as you practice the Minute Meditation. You will have thoughts; the practice is not about having no thoughts. It is about learning to being aware when you *are* dialoguing with those thoughts and gently returning to the silent aware-ness of your Spiritual Center *area*.

Do not concern yourself with do-ing it "right." If you are sitting for one minute twice a day, if, when thoughts or emotions arise, you lovingly return again and again to the silent aware-ness of your Spiritual Center *area*, then you are doing what is necessary. Be flexible.

Flexibility gives you the freedom to adjust to new routines. An active lifestyle requires flexibility: any change to a routine can create resistance. All too often, you may be attached to a particular schedule, time, or place. You may want everything to be the same day after day. In most situations, this might seem ideal.

Developing flexibility in your practice can lead to developing flexibility in all aspects of your life. Flexibility is a nurturing skill that will help you to be kinder to yourself. Go with what you have, wherever you are. You may want to sit for your first Minute Meditation practice of the day in the morning, and the second, during the afternoon or evening. If you find that fitting in a daily second practice is difficult—you can't find the time because of work, errands, children, and a million other things on your agenda that interfere — this is understandable.

Here's a suggestion: you do go to the bathroom sometime during your busy day, right? Stay on the John for an extra minute. It's that easy. Your friend, John, can be very helpful. In fact, John may become your *best* friend!

There is a silence within you that is so deafening that it can be heard. You may realize a silent voice that speaks to you when resting with the awareness of your Spiritual Center area. You may come to hear this silent voice more easily than any voice in this world. The silence is a timeless graced-gift of your nature. Penetrate it, and you are it.

8

Obstacles
Stepping Stones

As you practice meditation, you may realize that the mind finds a way to distract you from becoming aware of your Spiritual Center area. The mind is an expert at creating obstacles during a silent meditation practice. A meditation practice may turn obstacles into stepping stones that lead to the blessed peace within. The following are a few of the obstacles that the mind may revel in. Your awareness of them may shorten their lifespan.

Obstacles:

1. *Alone - Lonely*

As you progress with the practice, you may feel a sense of discomfort and loneliness because you may think of it as being alone. There is a difference between alone and lonely. Both have in common the inner message *"one"* (al*one* and l*one*ly). Alone rests in the "One." Lonely seeks the One. This world has so many tempting attractions to chase. You may, at times, do anything not to stay home alone.

When you are attached to a separate sense of a personal self, you experience a separate existence. You experience a sense of being lonely. Loneliness seeks a more profound presence of your nature, the Oneness.

Alone and lonely are no longer obstacles once you are no longer drawn to the background noise and chatter in your home environment. When you live with the quiet, you may come closer to realizing your true nature—the inner and the outer merge in a calm, peaceful environment. An environment where loneliness does not exist and being alone is restful, not restless.

2. *Attention*

Attention is your interest "instantly" alerted by the rising of thoughts, senses, or sense impressions (acting as stimuli) within your consciousness. The state of an object of interest holding your attention is called attentive concentration. Attention becomes an obstacle when it attaches you to thought, emotion, or sense-impression.

Attention is the mind's most devious obstacle. It is the easiest for the mind to use during silent meditation practice. Your attention is immediately attracted to whatever appears within your conscious mind. As your attention is drawn, it may seem to have a will of its own.

You subject yourself to suffering, pain, or pleasure by attending to or attaching emotions to the conditioned sense impressions or rising thoughts. It is your attracted interest that holds your attention. The greater the attraction, the greater chance the attention may become an obstacle. Thoughts and sense impressions do serve a purpose on this planet, when not practicing silent meditation. They allow a conscious flexible exploration of rising thoughts and sensations that may contribute to creativity, ideas, or resolutions.

As you continue the Minute Meditation practice, attention obstacles may gradually decrease. You may have a greater awareness of your spiritual nature. You have a choice over which thoughts and sensations you engage, act upon, or let go. You are in charge. This is interior freedom.

3. *Complacency*

You may become satisfied with your realized spiritual unfoldment. Complacency becomes an obstacle when you have lulled yourself into the false belief that you have surrendered enough. When your spiritual progress is at its smoothest, your boat may rock, and the complacency temptation will rise. Understanding why your boat should be rocked during what appears as smooth sailing may be challenging.

Complacency often invites a stiff-necked resistant response to an inner or outer nudge to take another step on the straight and narrow path. The practice takes you beyond, into turbulent deep waters. A struggle with temptation has the capacity to make you stronger, more convicted. Yours is a spiritual nature with many facets. The willingness to embrace the difficulties of yet another unknown facet of your spiritual nature allows a realized transition to be a more welcomed one.

4. *Greener Pastures*

You may be one who believes the grass is greener just beyond your own practice. It is difficult to remain faithful to your practice and progress if you have only one eye on where you are and the other on seeking greener pastures. In this world, greener pastures may appear one day and fade the next. Where you are is where the grass is the greenest. If you are tempted to other pastures, the grass will be just as green, no greener. This is a world of many pastures.

You could easily wander from one pasture to the next. The greener pasture that you seek is the one you are standing in, and with maintenance, the greener *it* becomes. The green pastures do not change. You do. The brilliance is within you. Stay with your practice.

5. *Internal Dialogue*

In meditation practice, internal dialogue is a conditioned response to rising thoughts or sense impressions (hearing, touch, sight, taste, and smell). It is the busy work of the mind. Internal dialogue is an obstacle that produces no benefit. It sidetracks and stalls a silent meditation practice. When your attention is attracted to rising thoughts, emotions, or senses, an internal dialogue may begin. Dialoguing is an obstacle that interferes with the immediacy of consciously returning to the awareness of your Spiritual Center area. Dialoguing negates the present moment of silence.

Internal dialogue deals primarily with memories or future expectations (planning). Neither memories of the past nor expectations of the future exist in the present. When a memory rises with an attached emotion (positive or negative), dialoguing recreates the event as if it were happening in the present. Such indulgence serves no useful purpose.

Not dialoguing is an essential tool in the purification process. Choosing not to dialogue internally with the attractions of this world, within the Minute Meditation practice or your daily life, may contribute to greater emotional stability. Not dialoguing with rising thoughts or memories is essential. If you do *not* dialogue with rising thoughts, emotions, sensations, and images, they will *not* become obstacles – they will fade.

~~

The Minute Meditation practice establishes you with unconditional, non-judgmental love emanating within your consciousness. You do not need to get upset with any obstacle or whatever rises within your consciousness. Just renew your priority and continue your meditation practice.

Your thought, word, and deed have a ripple effect. Whether you are near or far from the consciousness of individuals, the ripple effect of your thought, word, or deed may have a positive or negative influence. An act of kindness – or a malicious act – multiplies. Be aware if you think one thing but say another. Your thoughts, as well as your spoken words, vibrate, and go forth. Be faithful to your practice, and keep your actions gentle. Think twice before you speak and three times before you act. What you send out by the spoken word or thought will surely return to sender.

9

SUPPORTS
And
TOOLS
Helpful Suggestions

The following are a few helpful suggestions for your meditation practice. Work with the ones you are most comfortable with during meditation.

SUPPORTS:

1. Sitting

Sit in a comfortable position during silent meditation practice. Sitting may be on a couch, chair, or floor. If you practice sitting on a chair, you may choose to have a chair with arms on it for safety. Keep your head and chin relaxed and your hands on your lap or sides.

Sitting in the same area of your home or place of practice may facilitate comfort with your practice. However, the practice may be done anywhere your safety is not at risk. Sit still during your practice. If discomfort rises, slowly and quietly adjust your posture. Any movement while you are practicing should be performed in very slow motion. The less you disturb your vibrating energy, the better.

If you wish to stop your practice, stop. Do not force yourself to practice any particular length of time. Allow the time you practice to increase naturally. Be patient and gentle with your silent practice. Your determined purpose of sitting may form the sitting habit and allow you more easily to practice.

You are always encouraged to practice in a sitting position. If, for health reasons, you cannot sit, then, of course, lie down. However, guard against falling asleep. Remember, a fool goes to sleep, and a fool wakes up. You are practicing a silent meditation to wake up, not to take a nap.

Take a moment to readjust to your immediate environment at the end of your practice. Always get up carefully and slowly from your practic-ing position. If you wish, you may use a shawl. A shawl's purpose is to allow you to turn within more easily.

2. Time

Time is relative to this plane of opposites. When you first begin a silent meditation practice, you start with a minute twice a day. It is not necessary to intentionally place strict time limits on your silent practice. Allow your practice to expand itself naturally.

This allows your mind and body to naturally adjust to sitting. You do not want to judge your practice periods by length. Longer is not better or shorter worse. The critical issue is to do the practice twice a day. One minute is an eternity with the silence of awareness.

Your sitting will eventually become a habit. The time necessary for your practice will become established and comfortable. There never is a need to force your practice time. If you are restless or uncomfortable, get up and return to the practice at another time when you are at ease.

~~

3. Humor

As you are the one who ultimately benefits from forgiving, you are the one which also benefits from having a sense of humor. It is the gift that keeps on giving. It may help support your meditation practice. It may improve your relationships and your health. So, don't leave the house without it.

The best thing you could have on this earth plane, or develop, is a sense of humor. You do not want to leave this earth plane without one, and living well on this plane without one is impossible. Humor is the state of mind that allows you to appreciate the comical in times of stressful situations. Humor is one of the best relaxers. As many tend to do, you may begin to take yourself too seriously. Maintaining a sense of humor is essential for your mental and physical health.

Being serious at times, of course, may be necessary. However, you must not lose your sense of humor. Remember the great things surrounding you in times of sadness, such as nature's beauty. Learn to laugh at the apparent foolishness of this world. It may keep you from getting caught up in its illusions. Life is difficult enough, and it is next to impossible without an appreciation for the comical. Humor may lighten a serious situation and allow you to think more clearly.

At times, the inner journey may be a difficult one. But you are the only one who can lift you during these times. So, consider the foolish things you say and do. It should put a smile on your face and a sense of humor in your life.

~~

TOOLS

Tools are the aids on your inner path that may be used to assist you. These are some of the many tools of various kinds. What is considered sacred to you may not be to another. However, you may respect all available tools. It is your belief in any particular tool that matters. Tools may help guide you along your spiritual path.

Tools:
Books
Tapes
Stories
Symbols
Films
Shawls
Rituals
Cushions
Sacraments
Teachings

All tools serve to help your spiritual progress. Some may be of greater or lesser use at different stages of your practice. Tools should be approached with contemplative reverence. However, tools are about truth, not truth itself. The truth is who and what you are. It is not outside of your reality. Use whatever tool/s that you are drawn to and believe may help.

Guard against becoming attached to any tool. It is as if you have taken a boat to cross a river; once there, you do not carry the boat around on your head. You leave it for someone else to use.

Be grateful for its use; leave it behind when you are finished with any tool and move on. The critical thing to remember is that you never use any tool (a cushion and shawl are exceptions) when you are doing your meditation practice. Mixing your practice with tools or other practices will stall your spiritual progress. Don't do it. Your inner guidance needs no tool and can teach you all things directly. Your practice will meet your need in its own time. Supports and tools are useful, but you are all you ever need to practice meditation.

10

A
GIFT
A Bonus

Since you may be new at practicing meditation, I have a gift for you. It is a mini-exercise to add to your support system. It is a short, even easier practice. I think you will like it.

HAND-TO-CHEST EXERCISE

The Hand-to-Chest Exercise. may allow you to address difficult emotional situations, particularly if you need immediate help controlling your temper, fear, or excitement. There may be a time when your emotions are rising sky-high, and your energy is vibrating all over the place. The Hand-to-Chest Exercise may rescue you, instantly relieving stress and helping you keep your cool. That is a good thing!

The Exercise:

1. Whenever you are under emotional stress, anger, or a quick temper, quickly rest your hand upon your Spiritual Center *area*, the center of the chest, between the breasts.

2. Take a long, deep breath, and exhale slowly, relaxing your mind and body. Rest your attention on your hand (not on the awareness of your Spiritual Center area) with the silence of awareness. If necessary, repeat several times.

~~

That's it! It is short, quick, and easy. It is a *precious gift*. As you use the Hand-To-Chest Exercise, inner change may occur. Your Spiritual Center may transform your emotional energy. You may become calmer and settle down, allowing you to cope with difficulties. The Hand-to-Chest Exercise may bring you immediate relief.

Since you do not need to sit and close your eyes during this exercise, the Hand-to-Chest may be used at almost any time and anywhere. The exceptions are when your safety is at risk. You may use it alone, in a crowd, in a group, or on the go (not driving). The Hand-to-Chest Exercise takes only seconds. It may help you to be at your best under any circumstances.

Do not be fooled by the simplicity of this exercise. It may help bring immediate calm and restore your vibrating energy balance. Hands have always been used to heal, bless, and comfort. Your inner spiritual source may empower your hand as you rest it upon your Spiritual Center area. It is always available. Take advantage of it.

Summary

Meditation is good for you for many reasons: health, a balanced life, less stress, and interior cleansing. You are given a short easy meditation practice (the Minute Meditation), supporters, and tools to help you. Use them, and meditation will work for you.

Meditation presents you with new opportunities for your spiritual and practical growth. Practicing meditation may help you realize the power within your Spiritual Center so that you are guided to a life of balance, joy, peace, contentment, and full potential. Practice meditation. Start today; start now. You have everything you need: this book, the Spiritual Center, and you.

Accept the Minute Meditation challenge for eight weeks, and you may want to practice it for a lifetime. It is easy, yes, but it's profound. It's life-changing! Just one minute, twice a day, you may find that your life changes in ways you could not have imagined.

You may realize your spirituality and what is given to you; you may give. Who you are, you may share. Share the Minute Meditation with your family and friends. Will you do it? Are you up for it?

Most importantly, you will come away being aware that there is something more inside of you that you weren't aware existed. Your spirituality has been within you; it has always been there. You may consciously connect to and access it to realize your full potential.

Meditation *is* good for you. Practice the Minute Meditation, and you may find it has a life of *its* own. So, relax, enjoy, and let the practice *do* you.

TRANSLATOR

Carla R. Mancari is an author, translator, life guide, and teacher. She seeks to improve the self-confidence and self-esteem of individuals from all walks of life so that they can meet life's challenges. For more than 45 years, she has guided individuals in understanding life's spiritual principles, activities, and rising emotions in their private and daily lives. Carla is the recipient of the Christ Consciousness Meditation and the Minute Meditation. Although she had never attended high school and was labeled a retarded child, she attained two University degrees: a B.A. from the University of South Carolina in Columbia, South Carolina, and an MEd from South Carolina State University in Orangeburg, South Carolina. Carla studied at Brigham Young University and attended the School of the Americas in Switzerland.

Carla led a class action lawsuit in the United States Supreme Court to protect minorities' rights (Morton v. Mancari, 1973) and was a certified psychologist. She served in the United States Air Force. Traveling worldwide for many years, Carla studied with Christian, Hindu, and Buddhist masters. She was a guest on the Larry King Radio Show and a guest lecturer at various colleges, professional groups, book clubs, and at book signings. Carla gained national recognition when featured in *Good Housekeeping*, "The Education of Carla Mancari, 1969." It chronicled her life in 1967-68 when she was the first white woman to receive a Master's degree from the all-Black South Carolina State College in Orangeburg, South Carolina. She is the author of many books. Carla's greatest joy is helping individuals realize their self-worth, unique gifts/talents, and full potential, and wake up to their spiritual reality.

Books

Mancari, Carla R., *The Lessons: How to Understand Spiritual Principles, Spiritual Activities and Rising Emotions, A Comprehensive Collection.* Celestial Literary Group, 2026.

- - - *Christ Consciousness Meditation Practice: Pocket Size.* Celestial Literary Group, 2026.

- - - *Loneliness.* Celestial Literary Group, 2026.

- - - *Racism, Antisemitism+: A Disease of the Mind.* Celestial Literary Group, 2026.

- - - *The Christ Consciousness Meditation Teaching Guide.* Celestial Literary Group, 2026.

- - - *Metaphysical Questions with Answers from the Christ Consciousness.* Celestial Literary Group, 2026.

- - - *When Jesus Is the Guru: A Wayward Christian's Spiritual Walk.* Celestial Literary Group, 2010.

- - - *Eco-You: A Power of One, Improve Your Health, Improve Your Life.* Celestial Literary Group, 2019.

- - - *Walking on the Grass: A White Woman In A Black World.* Celestial Literary Group, 2016.

- - - *Abortion and The Bible: The Abortion Dilemma: A Scriptural Response, A Woman's Spirituality.* Celestial Literary Group, 2017.

- - - *Racism: The Pain of Invisibility.* Celestial Literary Group, 2017.

- - - *The Rising Emotions: Understanding and Mastering Them.* Celestial Literary Group, 2017.

- - - *The Mystical Path: The Serious Student.* Celestial Literary Group, 2017.

- - - *Spiritual Principles: Understanding, Realizing, and Living Them.* Celestial Literary Group, 2018.

- - - *Climate Change: Consciousness Change.* Celestial Literary Group, 2017.

- - - *Words: Locks On The Door or Keys To The Kingdom.* Celestial Literary Group, 2018.

- - - *Aging: Physical to the Mystical.* Celestial Literary Group, 2018.

- - - *Divine Love: Your Nature.* Celestial Literary Group, 2018.

- - - *The Lazarus Rising: The Kundalini – A Rising Dormant Energy.* Celestial Literary Group, 2018.

- - - *Depression: Hopelessness – A Disconnection.* Celestial Literary Group, 2018.

- - - *Jesus Christ: Teacher.* Celestial Literary Group, 2018.

- - - *The Mystical Surrender: Giving In.* Celestial Literary Group, 2018.

- - - *Death Ain't Dead: Empty Graves.* Celestial Literary Group, 2018.

- - - *Common Decency: Your DNA.* Celestial Literary Group, 2018.

- - - *Christians?: Common Decency.* Celestial Literary Group, 2018.

- - - *Beyond Buddhism: Meditations.* Celestial Literary Group, 2018.

- - - *Exit: Get Ready, Set, Go.* Celestial Literary Group, 2018.

- - - *Meditation: Good For You.* Celestial Literary Group, 2018.

- - - *How To Love "You": Begins with You.* Celestial Literary Group, 2018.

- - - *Consciousness: Yours.* Celestial Literary Group, 2018.

- - - *Suicide: Understanding It.* Celestial Literary Group, 2018.

- - - *Detachment: Realizations.* Celestial Literary Group, 2018.

- - - *Detachment: Christian.* Celestial Literary Group, 2018.

- - - *Sexual Abuse By The Church – Its Root, Coerced Celibacy.* Celestial Literary Group, 2018.

- - - *Guns and Guts: The Courage To Act.* Celestial Literary Group, 2018.

- - - *Jesus, The Way: A Mystical Understanding.* Celestial Literary Group, 2019.

- - - *Motivation: Self-Motivated.* Celestial Literary Group, 2019.

- - - *Totally Free: Is Killing Me.* Celestial Literary, Group, 2018.

- - - *A 30-Second Meditation For Teenagers.* Celestial Literary Group, 2018.

- - - *A 30-Second Meditation For Seniors.* Celestial Literary Group, 2017.

- - - *The Five Faces Of Love.* Celestial Literary Group, 2019.

- - - *Angel In The House.* Celestial Literary Group, 2019 (A Children's Book).

- - - *Put It In The Bible: Prayerful Requests.* Celestial Literary Group, 2019.

- - - *Hate: A Dark Emotion.* Celestial Literary Group, 2019.

- - - *Greed: It's Addictive.* Celestial Literary Group, 2019.

- - - *On Being Young: Choices.* Celestial Literary Group, 2019.

- - - *Gratitude: Expressed, Sincere.* Celestial Literary Group, 2019.

- - - *Humor: A Necessity.* Celestial Literary Group, 2019.

- - - *A Christian: Are You One?* Celestial Literary Group, 2019.

- - - *Habit: How To Switch Meditation Practices.* Celestial Literary Group, 2019.

- - - *Impeachment: Living On The Dark Side.* Celestial Literary Group, 2019.

- - - *The Jesus I Know.* Celestial Literary Group, 2019.

- - - *Grace: Spirit And Truth.* Celestial Literary Group, 2019.

- - - *Temptation.* Celestial Literary Group, 2019.

- - - *The Christian Journey: Teacher Student Relationship.* Celestial Literary Group, 2019.

- - - *The Beloved: Who Is The Beloved?* Celestial Literary Group, 2019.

- - - *What Now, Lord? Enlightenment.* Celestial Literary Group, 2019.

- - - *What If I Were Gay?* Celestial Literary Group, 2019.

- - - *Mother Mary: Mother of Jesus.* Celestial Literary Group, 2019.

- - - *I Remember America.* Celestial Literary Group, 2019.

- - - *The Overcoming: Jesus.* Celestial Literary Group, 2019.

- - - *When Faith Is Not Enough.* Celestial Literary Group, 2019.

- - - *The Plane of Opposites: The Work.* Celestial Literary Group, 2020.

- - - *Crisis.* Celestial Literary Group, 2020.

- - - *Grief: Gut-Wrenching Emotion.* Celestial Literary Group, 2020.

- - - *God.* Celestial Literary Group, 2020.

- - - *Regrets: Do You Have Any?* Celestial Literary Group, 2020.

- - - *1968, 1968,1968: The Mind of A Racist.* Celestial Literary Group, 2020.

- - - *Satan.* Celestial Literary Group, 2020.

- - - *Practice Practice: Meditation.* Celestial Literary Group, 2021.

- - - *Christians Without Jesus: Prodigal Son's Journey.* Celestial Literary Group, 2021.

- - - *From Here To There.* Celestial Literary Group, 2021.

- - - *An Awakening Path: Christian Spiritual Principles.* Celestial Literary Group, 2021.

- -.- *Holy Scriptures: Uplifting, Inspiring and Comforting.* Celestial Literary Group, 2021.

- - - *Male Female: The Split Soul.* Celestial Literary Group, 2021.

- - - *The Inner Message: Theological Mystical State.* Celestial Literary Group, 2021.

- - - *A Guide To Understanding Mind's Contents And Realizations.* Celestial Literary Group, 2021.

- - - *A Sister's Laughter: Oh! How I Miss It* Celestial Literary Group, 2021.

- - - *Churches: Are They Necessary?* Celestial Literary Group, 2021.

- - - *Metaphysical: Stories and Poems.* Celestial Literary Group, 2021.

- - - *Jesus, Jesus, Jesus.* Celestial Literary Group, 2021.

- - - *The Disciple and The Mystical Guide.* Celestial Literary Group, 2021.

- - - *The Holy Trinity: 1+1+1=1, No Mystery.* Celestial Literary Group, 2021.

- - - *Fear of Jesus: Why?.* Celestial Literary Group, 2021.

- - - *Symbols and Rituals: Christian.* Celestial Literary Group, 2021.

- - - *Christian Minute Meditation.* Celestial Literary Group, 2021.

- - - *Sin!.* Celestial Literary Group, 2021.

- - - *Compassion.* Celestial Literary Group, 2021.

- - - *Silence.* Celestial Literary Group, 2021.

- - - *The Spiritual Zone.* Celestial Literary Group, 2022.

- - - - *The Bible Scriptures: Mystical Understanding.* Celestial Literary Group, 2022.

- - - *Lead Us Not Into Temptation: The Lord's Prayer.* Celestial Literary Group, 2022.

- - - *Let's Talk About Jesus, Or Not.* Celestial Literary Group, 2022.

- - - *For The Love of Jesus: Come Back To Your Church.* Celestial Literary Group, 2022.

- - - *Abortion, When Life Does Not Begin! Exodus 21:22-25.* Celestial Literary Group, 2022.

- - - *Morton vs. Mancari: A Plaintiff's Response: How An Average Joe (woman) Landed In The US Supreme Court.* Celestial Literary Group, 2022.

- - - *Christian Spiritual Exercises: The Inner Journey.* Celestial Literary Group, 2023.

- - - *The Kingdom Of God – A Gift.* Celestial Literary Group, 2023.

- - - *An Expression of Love.* Celestial Literary Group, 2023.

- - - *Choices and Decisions On a Spiritual Journey.* Celestial Literary Group, 2024.

- - - *Love Your Enemies: How Can You Do That?.* Celestial Literary Group, 2024.

- - - *Outer Space and Inner Space Travel.* Celestial Literary Group, 2024.

- - - *God – Love: Poets Write About It.* Celestial Literary Group, 2024.

- - - *The Still Small Voice, You Can Hear It.* Celestial Literary Group, 2024.

- - - *The Resurrection: Rising Beyond Body Consciousness.* Celestial Literary Group, 2024.

- - - *Sexual Spiritual Intercourse: Oneness.* Celestial Literary Group, 2024.

- - - *Child Of God: In Spirit and Truth.* Celestial Literary Group, 2024.

- - - *"My Child," Blessed Mother Mary's.* Celestial Literary Group, 2024.

- - - *Strait Gate and Narrow Way: "Few There Be That Find It".* Celestial Literary Group, 2024.

- - - *Strait Gate and Narrow Way: "Few There Be That Find It", Pocket Size.* Celestial Literary Group, 2024.

- - - *The End Of The Beginning, Our Spiritual Journey.* Celestial Literary Group, 2024.

- - - *A Cat Story.* Celestial Literary Group, 2025.

Mancari, Carla. R. *and* Carpenter, Mary B. *Scriptural Reference For - The Lessons, A Comprehensive Collection.* Celestial Literary Group, 2026.

- - -*The Minute Meditation, Book 1: It Is Profound!* Celestial Literary Group, 2022.

- - -*The Minute Meditation, Book 2: Workbook, It Is Profound!.* The Celestial Literary Group, 2022.

- - - *The Minute Meditation, It Is Profound! Book 3: The Essentials.* Celestial Literary Group, 2022.

- - - *The Minute Meditation, It Is Profound! Book 4: A Diet For The Soul.* Celestial Literary Group, 2022.

- - - *The Minute Meditation, It Is Profound! Book 5: The Three of You, You Are Never Alone.* Celestial Literary Group, 2022.

- - - *The Minute Meditation, It Is Profound! Book 6: Pocket Size.* Celestial Literary Group, 2022.

- - - *The Minute Meditation, It Is Profound! Book 7 – Teaching Guide.* Celestial Literary Group, 2022.

- - - *The Minute Meditation, It Is Profound! Book 8 – The 4th Chakra.* Celestial Literary Group, 2026.

- - - *Spirituality: Yours.* Celestial Literary Group, 2021.

- - - *Dreams: States of Consciousness.* Celestial Literary Group, 2021.

- - - *A Christian Service With A Silent Christian Meditation.* Celestial Literary Group, 2024.

Casey-Martus, Sandra, and Mancari, Carla R. *The Lessons, How to Understand Spiritual Principles, Spiritual Activities and Rising Emotions, Lessons with Stories Along a Spiritual Journey.* Celestial Literary Group, 2026.

NOTES